MY 8-WEEK
intermittent
fasting
CHALLENGE

THIS BOOK BELONGS TO:

_____

Contents

How to Use
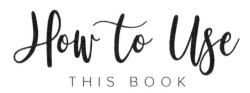

THIS BOOK

This book is designed to work with ANY fasting schedule. Whether you are testing different methods, or working your way up to longer fasting periods, this journal will allow you to plan and track any fasting schedule or to change it up as you go to fit what works best for you. If you take a break from fasting, you can pick up again any time with this undated tracker.

Take before pictures and fill out the before + after page. Write down what you are hoping to get out of fasting and what you want to accomplish.

Weekly Planning

Plan your week with the calendar page. Color code eating hours for the week vs fasting hours for the week. Draw lines through your planned sleeping hours. Your sleeping hours will overlap with fasting hours. Do not use heavy markers to avoid bleeding through the page. Gel pens and highlighters work fantastic as well as colored pencils or washi tape.

Daily Tracking

Each day has prompts to track your IF plan, sleep, water, food, exercise as well as a variety of other emotions and symptoms that can arise as a result of different fasting methods. Feel free to add other notes such as ketones, blood pressure, blood sugars, and data that is specific to your health goals in the journaling section.

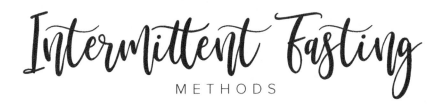
Intermittent Fasting

M E T H O D S

1 4 / 1 0   M E T H O D
Eat during a 10 hour window, fast during a 14 hour window. This is a great place to start transitioning from grazing to an IF lifestyle. This is a fasting method that can be done daily.

1 6 / 8   M E T H O D
Eat during an 8 hour window, fast during a 16 hour window. For example, only eat during the hours of noon to 8pm. This is a very popular IF schedule. You sleep during a good portion of the fast and it is simple to choose which meal to "skip" for the day. This fasting method can be done daily or only on certain days of the week.

2 0   H O U R   M E T H O D
Eat all of your calories for the day within a 4 hour window. For example, from 2pm-6pm.

2 4   H O U R   M E T H O D
This method should only be done once or twice per week. It is best to have your last meal (can be breakfast, lunch or dinner) and then not eat again until that same meal the next day. For example, if your last meal is dinner, don't eat again until dinner the next day.

3 6   H O U R   M E T H O D
You will fast for an entire day using this method. For example, you finish dinner on day 1 at 7pm and then skip all meals on day 2, not eating again until breakfast at 7am on day 3. This should only be done once per week.

5 / 2   M E T H O D
In this fasting method, you will eat normally for 5 days but on 2 non-consecutive days, you limit your caloric intake to 500.

A D F   M E T H O D
Alternate Day Fasting is when you pick any method above and practice it every other day.

Dos & Dont's

Be Sure To

- Drink plenty of water
- Eat healthy foods
- Get plenty of sleep
- Consider a trial fast to learn the difference between mental & physical hunger
- Break your fast gently with broth, lemon water, or fruit juices
- Listen to your body
- Deal with emotions that do not serve you anymore.

LISTEN TO YOUR BODY

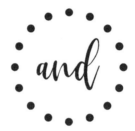

and

ADJUST YOUR PLAN IF NEEDED

Do Not

- Fast at all if you have a history of eating disorders or are pregnant / nursing.
- Binge eat during the eating hours
- Break the fast with a huge meal

Mental Hunger
WAYS TO FIGHT IT

As you begin your IF trials and schedule, you will learn the difference between MENTAL and PHYSICAL hunger. To help fight mental hunger:

- drink water
- eat protein
- physically distance yourself from the craving (don't have it in the house)
- sip tea
- go for a walk
- take a hot bath with epsom salt + lavendar oil
- exercise
- meditate / practice mindfulness
- brush your teeth and go to bed

Ask Yourself

- Am I hungry enough to eat a vegetable? If I'm not, it's probably not true hunger.
- Do I want to eat to fuel my body? Or am I looking for a sense of security?
- Is my stomach physically rumbling? Or am I feeling stressed or overwhelmed?
- Am I choosing nutritious foods? Or am I choosing comfort foods?

About Perfection

If you give in to a craving or eat when you didn't plan to, the worst thing you can do is throw in the towel. Falling off-plan is normal and happens especially with monthly hormonal changes. If you choose to eat a brownie, that does NOT mean you might as well eat the entire pan. A few bites is substantially better than the whole pan. Being perfect can never be maintained as a LIFESTYLE and trying to be increases your chance of failure. Plan to be flexible and when you give in, just move on.

Progress

Physical

DATE:								
WEIGHT								
CHEST								
WAIST (smallest point)								
WAIST (at belly button)								
HIPS								
THIGHS								
BICEP								

Psychological

DATE:								
HAPPY WITH BODY								
ENERGETIC								
STRONG								
SKILLED at portion control								
CAN DISCERN mental vs physical hunger								

HOW DO YOU FEEL ON A SCALE OF 1-10 (10 BEING HIGHEST)

. . . . .

THIS IS THE

beginning

OF

anything

YOU

want.

. . . . .

Planning

	S	M	T	W	T	F	S	NOTES
MIDNIGHT								....
1:00 AM								....
2:00 AM								....
3:00 AM								....
4:00 AM								....
5:00 AM								....
6:00 AM								....
7:00 AM								....
8:00 AM								....
9:00 AM								....
10:00 AM								....
11:00 AM								....
NOON								....
1:00 PM								....
2:00 PM								....
3:00 PM								....
4:00 PM								....
5:00 PM								....
6:00 PM								....
7:00 PM								....
8:00 PM								....
9:00 PM								....
10:00 PM								....
11:00 PM								....
MIDNIGHT								....
								....

EATING   FASTING   SLEEPING

plan your week
COLOR CODE YOUR HOURS

(J) (F) (M) (A) (M) (J) (J) (A) (S) (O) (N) (D)

| 1 | 2 | 3 | 4 | 5 | 6 | 7 | 8 | 9 | 10 | 11 | 12 | 13 | 14 | 15 | 16 |

| 17 | 18 | 19 | 20 | 21 | 22 | 23 | 24 | 25 | 26 | 27 | 28 | 29 | 30 | 31 | ♥ |

Fasting Day? YES / NO

FIRST BITE: _____   FASTING HOURS: _____

LAST BITE: _____   EATING HOURS: _____

Sleep

TO BED: _____   HOURS SLEPT: _____

WOKE UP: _____   QUALITY: _____

Food	Time	Note

Exercise	Time	Note

Habits

WATER   ⬠ ⬠ ⬠ ⬠ ⬠ ⬠ ⬠

ENERGY LEVEL 😄 😐 🙁

HUNGER 😄 😐 🙁

MENTAL STRENGTH 😄 😐 🙁

REGULARITY 😄 😐 🙁

MOOD 😄 😐 🙁

BRAIN CLARITY 😄 😐 🙁

Journaling

....

....

....

....

....

....

....

....

....

....

....

....

....

| J | F | M | A | M | J | J | A | S | O | N | D |

| 1 | 2 | 3 | 4 | 5 | 6 | 7 | 8 | 9 | 10 | 11 | 12 | 13 | 14 | 15 | 16 |
| 17 | 18 | 19 | 20 | 21 | 22 | 23 | 24 | 25 | 26 | 27 | 28 | 29 | 30 | 31 | ♥ |

Fasting Day? YES / NO

FIRST BITE: _____   FASTING HOURS: _____

LAST BITE: _____   EATING HOURS: _____

Sleep

TO BED: _____   HOURS SLEPT: _____

WOKE UP: _____   QUALITY: _____

Food	Time	Note

Exercise	Time	Note

Habits

WATER ⬡⬡⬡⬡⬡⬡⬡

ENERGY LEVEL ☺ 😐 ☹
HUNGER ☺ 😐 ☹
MENTAL STRENGTH ☺ 😐 ☹
REGULARITY ☺ 😐 ☹
MOOD ☺ 😐 ☹
BRAIN CLARITY ☺ 😐 ☹

Journaling

....
....
....
....
....
....
....
....
....
....
....
....
....

(J) (F) (M) (A) (M) (J) (J) (A) (S) (O) (N) (D)

1 2 3 4 5 6 7 8 9 10 11 12 13 14 15 16

17 18 19 20 21 22 23 24 25 26 27 28 29 30 31 ♥

Fasting Day? YES / NO

FIRST BITE: _____   FASTING HOURS: _____

LAST BITE: _____   EATING HOURS: _____

Sleep

TO BED: _____   HOURS SLEPT: _____

WOKE UP: _____   QUALITY: _____

Food	Time	Note

Exercise	Time	Note

Habits

WATER ⬡⬡⬡⬡⬡⬡⬡⬡

ENERGY LEVEL ☺ 😐 ☹
HUNGER ☺ 😐 ☹
MENTAL STRENGTH ☺ 😐 ☹
REGULARITY ☺ 😐 ☹
MOOD ☺ 😐 ☹
BRAIN CLARITY ☺ 😐 ☹

Journaling

....
....
....
....
....
....
....
....
....
....
....
....

Fasting Day? YES / NO

FIRST BITE: _____   FASTING HOURS: _____

LAST BITE: _____   EATING HOURS: _____

Sleep

TO BED: _____   HOURS SLEPT: _____

WOKE UP: _____   QUALITY: _____

Food	Time	Note

Exercise	Time	Note

Habits

WATER ⬦⬦⬦⬦⬦⬦⬦

ENERGY LEVEL ☺ 😐 ☹
HUNGER ☺ 😐 ☹
MENTAL STRENGTH ☺ 😐 ☹
REGULARITY ☺ 😐 ☹
MOOD ☺ 😐 ☹
BRAIN CLARITY ☺ 😐 ☹

Journaling

....
....
....
....
....
....
....
....
....
....
....
....

$\left(\mathcal{J}\right)$ $\left(\mathcal{F}\right)$ $\left(\mathcal{M}\right)$ $\left(\mathcal{A}\right)$ $\left(\mathcal{M}\right)$ $\left(\mathcal{J}\right)$ $\left(\mathcal{J}\right)$ $\left(\mathcal{A}\right)$ $\left(\mathcal{S}\right)$ $\left(\mathcal{O}\right)$ $\left(\mathcal{N}\right)$ $\left(\mathcal{D}\right)$

1 2 3 4 5 6 7 8 9 10 11 12 13 14 15 16

17 18 19 20 21 22 23 24 25 26 27 28 29 30 31 ❤

Fasting Day? YES / NO

FIRST BITE: _____   FASTING HOURS: _____

LAST BITE: _____   EATING HOURS: _____

Sleep

TO BED: _____   HOURS SLEPT: _____

WOKE UP: _____   QUALITY: _____

Food	Time	Note

Exercise	Time	Note

Habits

WATER ⬡ ⬡ ⬡ ⬡ ⬡ ⬡ ⬡ ⬡

ENERGY LEVEL 😃 😐 🙁
HUNGER 😃 😐 🙁
MENTAL STRENGTH 😃 😐 🙁
REGULARITY 😃 😐 🙁
MOOD 😃 😐 🙁
BRAIN CLARITY 😃 😐 🙁

Journaling

....
....
....
....
....
....
....
....
....
....
....
....
....

(J) (F) (M) (A) (M) (J) (J) (A) (S) (O) (N) (D)

| 1 | 2 | 3 | 4 | 5 | 6 | 7 | 8 | 9 | 10 | 11 | 12 | 13 | 14 | 15 | 16 |

| 17 | 18 | 19 | 20 | 21 | 22 | 23 | 24 | 25 | 26 | 27 | 28 | 29 | 30 | 31 | ♥ |

Fasting Day? YES / NO

FIRST BITE: _____   FASTING HOURS: _____

LAST BITE: _____   EATING HOURS: _____

Sleep

TO BED: _____   HOURS SLEPT: _____

WOKE UP: _____   QUALITY: _____

Food	Time	Note

Exercise	Time	Note

Habits

WATER ⬡ ⬡ ⬡ ⬡ ⬡ ⬡ ⬡

ENERGY LEVEL 😄 😐 ☹️
HUNGER 😄 😐 ☹️
MENTAL STRENGTH 😄 😐 ☹️
REGULARITY 😄 😐 ☹️
MOOD 😄 😐 ☹️
BRAIN CLARITY 😄 😐 ☹️

Journaling

....
....
....
....
....
....
....
....
....
....
....
....

J	F	M	A	M	J	J	A	S	O	N	D

1	2	3	4	5	6	7	8	9	10	11	12	13	14	15	16
17	18	19	20	21	22	23	24	25	26	27	28	29	30	31	❤

Fasting Day? YES / NO

FIRST BITE: _____   FASTING HOURS: _____

LAST BITE: _____   EATING HOURS: _____

Sleep

TO BED: _____   HOURS SLEPT: _____

WOKE UP: _____   QUALITY: _____

Food	Time	Note

Exercise	Time	Note

Habits

WATER   ◊ ◊ ◊ ◊ ◊ ◊ ◊ ◊

ENERGY LEVEL ☺ 😐 ☹
HUNGER ☺ 😐 ☹
MENTAL STRENGTH ☺ 😐 ☹
REGULARITY ☺ 😐 ☹
MOOD ☺ 😐 ☹
BRAIN CLARITY ☺ 😐 ☹

Journaling

....
....
....
....
....
....
....
....
....
....
....
....
....

Planning

	S	M	T	W	T	F	S	NOTES
MIDNIGHT								
1:00 AM								
2:00 AM								
3:00 AM								
4:00 AM								
5:00 AM								
6:00 AM								
7:00 AM								
8:00 AM								
9:00 AM								
10:00 AM								
11:00 AM								
NOON								
1:00 PM								
2:00 PM								
3:00 PM								
4:00 PM								
5:00 PM								
6:00 PM								
7:00 PM								
8:00 PM								
9:00 PM								
10:00 PM								
11:00 PM								
MIDNIGHT								

EATING FASTING SLEEPING

plan your week
COLOR CODE YOUR HOURS

Fasting Day? YES / NO

FIRST BITE: _____   FASTING HOURS: _____

LAST BITE: _____   EATING HOURS: _____

Sleep

TO BED: _____   HOURS SLEPT: _____

WOKE UP: _____   QUALITY: _____

Food	Time	Note

Exercise	Time	Note

Habits

WATER ○ ○ ○ ○ ○ ○ ○

ENERGY LEVEL 🙂 😐 🙁
HUNGER 🙂 😐 🙁
MENTAL STRENGTH 🙂 😐 🙁
REGULARITY 🙂 😐 🙁
MOOD 🙂 😐 🙁
BRAIN CLARITY 🙂 😐 🙁

Journaling

....
....
....
....
....
....
....
....
....
....
....
....
....

Fasting Day? YES / NO

FIRST BITE: _____   FASTING HOURS: _____

LAST BITE: _____   EATING HOURS: _____

Sleep

TO BED: _____   HOURS SLEPT: _____

WOKE UP: _____   QUALITY: _____

Food	Time	Note

Exercise	Time	Note

Habits

WATER ⬦⬦⬦⬦⬦⬦⬦

ENERGY LEVEL ☺ 😐 ☹
HUNGER ☺ 😐 ☹
MENTAL STRENGTH ☺ 😐 ☹
REGULARITY ☺ 😐 ☹
MOOD ☺ 😐 ☹
BRAIN CLARITY ☺ 😐 ☹

Journaling

....
....
....
....
....
....
....
....
....
....
....
....
....

Fasting Day? YES / NO

FIRST BITE: _____   FASTING HOURS: _____

LAST BITE: _____   EATING HOURS: _____

Sleep

TO BED: _____   HOURS SLEPT: _____

WOKE UP: _____   QUALITY: _____

Food	Time	Note

Exercise	Time	Note

Habits

WATER ⬡⬡⬡⬡⬡⬡⬡⬡

ENERGY LEVEL ☺ ☺ ☹
HUNGER ☺ ☺ ☹
MENTAL STRENGTH ☺ ☺ ☹
REGULARITY ☺ ☺ ☹
MOOD ☺ ☺ ☹
BRAIN CLARITY ☺ ☺ ☹

Journaling

....
....
....
....
....
....
....
....
....
....
....
....
....

Fasting Day? YES / NO

FIRST BITE: _____   FASTING HOURS: _____

LAST BITE: _____   EATING HOURS: _____

Sleep

TO BED: _____   HOURS SLEPT: _____

WOKE UP: _____   QUALITY: _____

Food	Time	Note

Exercise	Time	Note

Habits

WATER ⬦ ⬦ ⬦ ⬦ ⬦ ⬦ ⬦

ENERGY LEVEL ☺ 😐 ☹
HUNGER ☺ 😐 ☹
MENTAL STRENGTH ☺ 😐 ☹
REGULARITY ☺ 😐 ☹
MOOD ☺ 😐 ☹
BRAIN CLARITY ☺ 😐 ☹

Journaling

....
....
....
....
....
....
....
....
....
....
....
....
....

Fasting Day?   YES / NO

FIRST BITE: _____   FASTING HOURS: _____

LAST BITE: _____   EATING HOURS: _____

Sleep

TO BED: _____   HOURS SLEPT: _____

WOKE UP: _____   QUALITY: _____

Food	Time	Note

Exercise	Time	Note

Habits

WATER ⬠ ⬠ ⬠ ⬠ ⬠ ⬠ ⬠

ENERGY LEVEL 🙂 😐 🙁
HUNGER 🙂 😐 🙁
MENTAL STRENGTH 🙂 😐 🙁
REGULARITY 🙂 😐 🙁
MOOD 🙂 😐 🙁
BRAIN CLARITY 🙂 😐 🙁

Journaling

....
....
....
....
....
....
....
....
....
....
....
....
....

Fasting Day? YES / NO

FIRST BITE: _____   FASTING HOURS: _____

LAST BITE: _____   EATING HOURS: _____

Sleep

TO BED: _____   HOURS SLEPT: _____

WOKE UP: _____   QUALITY: _____

Food	Time	Note

Exercise	Time	Note

Habits

WATER ⬡⬡⬡⬡⬡⬡⬡⬡

ENERGY LEVEL ☺ 😐 ☹
HUNGER ☺ 😐 ☹
MENTAL STRENGTH ☺ 😐 ☹
REGULARITY ☺ 😐 ☹
MOOD ☺ 😐 ☹
BRAIN CLARITY ☺ 😐 ☹

Journaling

....
....
....
....
....
....
....
....
....
....
....
....
....

Fasting Day? YES / NO

FIRST BITE: _____   FASTING HOURS: _____

LAST BITE: _____   EATING HOURS: _____

Sleep

TO BED: _____   HOURS SLEPT: _____

WOKE UP: _____   QUALITY: _____

Food	Time	Note

Exercise	Time	Note

Habits

WATER ⬡⬡⬡⬡⬡⬡⬡

ENERGY LEVEL ☺ 😐 ☹
HUNGER ☺ 😐 ☹
MENTAL STRENGTH ☺ 😐 ☹
REGULARITY ☺ 😐 ☹
MOOD ☺ 😐 ☹
BRAIN CLARITY ☺ 😐 ☹

Journaling

....
....
....
....
....
....
....
....
....
....
....
....
....

Planning

	S	M	T	W	T	F	S	NOTES
MIDNIGHT								
1:00 AM								
2:00 AM								
3:00 AM								
4:00 AM								
5:00 AM								
6:00 AM								
7:00 AM								
8:00 AM								
9:00 AM								
10:00 AM								
11:00 AM								
NOON								
1:00 PM								
2:00 PM								
3:00 PM								
4:00 PM								
5:00 PM								
6:00 PM								
7:00 PM								
8:00 PM								
9:00 PM								
10:00 PM								
11:00 PM								
MIDNIGHT								

EATING   FASTING   SLEEPING

plan your week
COLOR CODE YOUR HOURS

(J) (F) (M) (A) (M) (J) (J) (A) (S) (O) (N) (D)

| 1 | 2 | 3 | 4 | 5 | 6 | 7 | 8 | 9 | 10 | 11 | 12 | 13 | 14 | 15 | 16 |

| 17 | 18 | 19 | 20 | 21 | 22 | 23 | 24 | 25 | 26 | 27 | 28 | 29 | 30 | 31 | ♥ |

Fasting Day? YES / NO

FIRST BITE: _____   FASTING HOURS: _____

LAST BITE: _____   EATING HOURS: _____

Sleep

TO BED: _____   HOURS SLEPT: _____

WOKE UP: _____   QUALITY: _____

Food	Time	Note

Exercise	Time	Note

Habits

WATER   ⬡ ⬡ ⬡ ⬡ ⬡ ⬡ ⬡

ENERGY LEVEL   😃 😐 ☹️
HUNGER   😃 😐 ☹️
MENTAL STRENGTH   😃 😐 ☹️
REGULARITY   😃 😐 ☹️
MOOD   😃 😐 ☹️
BRAIN CLARITY   😃 😐 ☹️

Journaling

....
....
....
....
....
....
....
....
....
....
....
....
....

Fasting Day? YES / NO

FIRST BITE: _____   FASTING HOURS: _____

LAST BITE: _____   EATING HOURS: _____

Sleep

TO BED: _____   HOURS SLEPT: _____

WOKE UP: _____   QUALITY: _____

Food	Time	Note

Exercise	Time	Note

Habits

WATER ⬯ ⬯ ⬯ ⬯ ⬯ ⬯ ⬯

ENERGY LEVEL ☺ 😐 ☹
HUNGER ☺ 😐 ☹
MENTAL STRENGTH ☺ 😐 ☹
REGULARITY ☺ 😐 ☹
MOOD ☺ 😐 ☹
BRAIN CLARITY ☺ 😐 ☹

Journaling

....
....
....
....
....
....
....
....
....
....
....
....

J F M A M J J A S O N D

| 1 | 2 | 3 | 4 | 5 | 6 | 7 | 8 | 9 | 10 | 11 | 12 | 13 | 14 | 15 | 16 |

| 17 | 18 | 19 | 20 | 21 | 22 | 23 | 24 | 25 | 26 | 27 | 28 | 29 | 30 | 31 | ♥ |

Fasting Day? YES / NO

FIRST BITE: _____   FASTING HOURS: _____

LAST BITE: _____   EATING HOURS: _____

Sleep

TO BED: _____   HOURS SLEPT: _____

WOKE UP: _____   QUALITY: _____

Food	Time	Note

Exercise	Time	Note

Habits

WATER ⬦⬦⬦⬦⬦⬦⬦⬦

ENERGY LEVEL ☺ 😐 ☹
HUNGER ☺ 😐 ☹
MENTAL STRENGTH ☺ 😐 ☹
REGULARITY ☺ 😐 ☹
MOOD ☺ 😐 ☹
BRAIN CLARITY ☺ 😐 ☹

Journaling

....
....
....
....
....
....
....
....
....
....
....
....

(J) (F) (M) (A) (M) (J) (J) (A) (S) (O) (N) (D)

| 1 | 2 | 3 | 4 | 5 | 6 | 7 | 8 | 9 | 10 | 11 | 12 | 13 | 14 | 15 | 16 |

| 17 | 18 | 19 | 20 | 21 | 22 | 23 | 24 | 25 | 26 | 27 | 28 | 29 | 30 | 31 | ♥ |

Fasting Day? YES / NO

FIRST BITE: _____   FASTING HOURS: _____

LAST BITE: _____   EATING HOURS: _____

Sleep

TO BED: _____   HOURS SLEPT: _____

WOKE UP: _____   QUALITY: _____

Food	Time	Note

Exercise	Time	Note

Habits

WATER ◊◊◊◊◊◊◊

ENERGY LEVEL ☺ ☺ ☹
HUNGER ☺ ☺ ☹
MENTAL STRENGTH ☺ ☺ ☹
REGULARITY ☺ ☺ ☹
MOOD ☺ ☺ ☹
BRAIN CLARITY ☺ ☺ ☹

Journaling

....
....
....
....
....
....
....
....
....
....
....
....
....

Fasting Day? YES / NO

FIRST BITE: _____   FASTING HOURS: _____

LAST BITE: _____   EATING HOURS: _____

Sleep

TO BED: _____   HOURS SLEPT: _____

WOKE UP: _____   QUALITY: _____

Food	Time	Note

Exercise	Time	Note

Habits

WATER ⬡⬡⬡⬡⬡⬡⬡

ENERGY LEVEL ☺ 😐 ☹
HUNGER ☺ 😐 ☹
MENTAL STRENGTH ☺ 😐 ☹
REGULARITY ☺ 😐 ☹
MOOD ☺ 😐 ☹
BRAIN CLARITY ☺ 😐 ☹

Journaling

....
....
....
....
....
....
....
....
....
....
....
....
....
....

J F M A M J J A S O N D

| 1 | 2 | 3 | 4 | 5 | 6 | 7 | 8 | 9 | 10 | 11 | 12 | 13 | 14 | 15 | 16 |

17 18 19 20 21 22 23 24 25 26 27 28 29 30 31 ♥

Fasting Day? YES / NO

FIRST BITE: _____   FASTING HOURS: _____

LAST BITE: _____   EATING HOURS: _____

Sleep

TO BED: _____   HOURS SLEPT: _____

WOKE UP: _____   QUALITY: _____

Food	Time	Note

Exercise	Time	Note

Habits

WATER ⬡ ⬡ ⬡ ⬡ ⬡ ⬡ ⬡

ENERGY LEVEL 😃 😐 🙁
HUNGER 😃 😐 🙁
MENTAL STRENGTH 😃 😐 🙁
REGULARITY 😃 😐 🙁
MOOD 😃 😐 🙁
BRAIN CLARITY 😃 😐 🙁

Journaling

....
....
....
....
....
....
....
....
....
....
....
....
....

Fasting Day? YES / NO

FIRST BITE: _____   FASTING HOURS: _____

LAST BITE: _____   EATING HOURS: _____

Sleep

TO BED: _____   HOURS SLEPT: _____

WOKE UP: _____   QUALITY: _____

Food	Time	Note

Exercise	Time	Note

Habits

WATER ◊ ◊ ◊ ◊ ◊ ◊ ◊ ◊

ENERGY LEVEL ☺ ☺ ☹
HUNGER ☺ ☺ ☹
MENTAL STRENGTH ☺ ☺ ☹
REGULARITY ☺ ☺ ☹
MOOD ☺ ☺ ☹
BRAIN CLARITY ☺ ☺ ☹

Journaling

....
....
....
....
....
....
....
....
....
....
....
....
....

Planning

	S	M	T	W	T	F	S	NOTES
MIDNIGHT								. . . .
1:00 AM								. . . .
2:00 AM								. . . .
3:00 AM								. . . .
4:00 AM								. . . .
5:00 AM								. . . .
6:00 AM								. . . .
7:00 AM								. . . .
8:00 AM								
9:00 AM								
10:00 AM								. . . .
11:00 AM								. . . .
NOON								. . . .
1:00 PM								. . . .
2:00 PM								. . . .
3:00 PM								. . . .
4:00 PM								. . . .
5:00 PM								. . . .
6:00 PM								. . . .
7:00 PM								. . . .
8:00 PM								
9:00 PM								
10:00 PM								. . . .
11:00 PM								. . . .
MIDNIGHT								. . . .

☐ EATING   ☐ FASTING   ◩ SLEEPING

plan your week
COLOR CODE YOUR HOURS

Fasting Day? YES / NO

FIRST BITE: _____   FASTING HOURS: _____

LAST BITE: _____   EATING HOURS: _____

Sleep

TO BED: _____   HOURS SLEPT: _____

WOKE UP: _____   QUALITY: _____

Food	Time	Note

Exercise	Time	Note

Habits

WATER ◊◊◊◊◊◊◊

ENERGY LEVEL ☺ 😐 ☹
HUNGER ☺ 😐 ☹
MENTAL STRENGTH ☺ 😐 ☹
REGULARITY ☺ 😐 ☹
MOOD ☺ 😐 ☹
BRAIN CLARITY ☺ 😐 ☹

Journaling

....
....
....
....
....
....
....
....
....
....
....
....
....

Fasting Day? YES / NO

FIRST BITE: _____   FASTING HOURS: _____

LAST BITE: _____   EATING HOURS: _____

Sleep

TO BED: _____   HOURS SLEPT: _____

WOKE UP: _____   QUALITY: _____

Food	Time	Note

Exercise	Time	Note

Habits

WATER ⬠⬠⬠⬠⬠⬠⬠⬠

ENERGY LEVEL 😊 😐 🙁
HUNGER 😊 😐 🙁
MENTAL STRENGTH 😊 😐 🙁
REGULARITY 😊 😐 🙁
MOOD 😊 😐 🙁
BRAIN CLARITY 😊 😐 🙁

Journaling

....
....
....
....
....
....
....
....
....
....
....
....
....

Fasting Day? YES / NO

FIRST BITE: _____   FASTING HOURS: _____

LAST BITE: _____   EATING HOURS: _____

Sleep

TO BED: _____   HOURS SLEPT: _____

WOKE UP: _____   QUALITY: _____

Food	Time	Note

Exercise	Time	Note

Habits

WATER ⬡⬡⬡⬡⬡⬡⬡⬡

ENERGY LEVEL 😊 😐 ☹️
HUNGER 😊 😐 ☹️
MENTAL STRENGTH 😊 😐 ☹️
REGULARITY 😊 😐 ☹️
MOOD 😊 😐 ☹️
BRAIN CLARITY 😊 😐 ☹️

Journaling

....
....
....
....
....
....
....
....
....
....
....
....
....

Fasting Day? YES / NO

FIRST BITE: _____   FASTING HOURS: _____

LAST BITE: _____   EATING HOURS: _____

Sleep

TO BED: _____   HOURS SLEPT: _____

WOKE UP: _____   QUALITY: _____

Food	Time	Note

Exercise	Time	Note

Habits

WATER   ◇ ◇ ◇ ◇ ◇ ◇ ◇

ENERGY LEVEL ☺ ☻ ☹
HUNGER ☺ ☻ ☹
MENTAL STRENGTH ☺ ☻ ☹
REGULARITY ☺ ☻ ☹
MOOD ☺ ☻ ☹
BRAIN CLARITY ☺ ☻ ☹

Journaling

....
....
....
....
....
....
....
....
....
....
....
....

Fasting Day? YES / NO

FIRST BITE: _____   FASTING HOURS: _____

LAST BITE: _____   EATING HOURS: _____

Sleep

TO BED: _____   HOURS SLEPT: _____

WOKE UP: _____   QUALITY: _____

Food	Time	Note

Exercise	Time	Note

Habits

WATER   ◇ ◇ ◇ ◇ ◇ ◇ ◇ ◇

ENERGY LEVEL 🙂 😐 🙁
HUNGER 🙂 😐 🙁
MENTAL STRENGTH 🙂 😐 🙁
REGULARITY 🙂 😐 🙁
MOOD 🙂 😐 🙁
BRAIN CLARITY 🙂 😐 🙁

Journaling

....
....
....
....
....
....
....
....
....
....
....
....

Fasting Day? YES / NO

FIRST BITE: _____   FASTING HOURS: _____

LAST BITE: _____   EATING HOURS: _____

Sleep

TO BED: _____   HOURS SLEPT: _____

WOKE UP: _____   QUALITY: _____

Food	Time	Note

Exercise	Time	Note

Habits

WATER ○○○○○○○

ENERGY LEVEL ☺ 😐 ☹
HUNGER ☺ 😐 ☹
MENTAL STRENGTH ☺ 😐 ☹
REGULARITY ☺ 😐 ☹
MOOD ☺ 😐 ☹
BRAIN CLARITY ☺ 😐 ☹

Journaling

....
....
....
....
....
....
....
....
....
....
....
....
....
....

Fasting Day? YES / NO

FIRST BITE: _____   FASTING HOURS: _____

LAST BITE: _____   EATING HOURS: _____

Sleep

TO BED: _____   HOURS SLEPT: _____

WOKE UP: _____   QUALITY: _____

Food	Time	Note

Exercise	Time	Note

Habits

WATER   ⬭ ⬭ ⬭ ⬭ ⬭ ⬭ ⬭

ENERGY LEVEL   😃 😐 ☹️
HUNGER   😃 😐 ☹️
MENTAL STRENGTH   😃 😐 ☹️
REGULARITY   😃 😐 ☹️
MOOD   😃 😐 ☹️
BRAIN CLARITY   😃 😐 ☹️

Journaling

....
....
....
....
....
....
....
....
....
....
....
....

Planning

	S	M	T	W	T	F	S	NOTES
MIDNIGHT								....
1:00 AM								....
2:00 AM								....
3:00 AM								....
4:00 AM								....
5:00 AM								....
6:00 AM								....
7:00 AM								....
8:00 AM								....
9:00 AM								....
10:00 AM								....
11:00 AM								....
NOON								....
1:00 PM								....
2:00 PM								....
3:00 PM								....
4:00 PM								....
5:00 PM								....
6:00 PM								....
7:00 PM								....
8:00 PM								....
9:00 PM								....
10:00 PM								....
11:00 PM								....
MIDNIGHT								....
								....

☐ EATING   ☐ FASTING   ☒ SLEEPING

plan your week
COLOR CODE YOUR HOURS

Fasting Day? YES / NO

FIRST BITE: _____   FASTING HOURS: _____

LAST BITE: _____   EATING HOURS: _____

Sleep

TO BED: _____   HOURS SLEPT: _____

WOKE UP: _____   QUALITY: _____

Food	Time	Note

Exercise	Time	Note

Habits

WATER ⬡⬡⬡⬡⬡⬡⬡

ENERGY LEVEL 😃 😐 ☹️
HUNGER 😃 😐 ☹️
MENTAL STRENGTH 😃 😐 ☹️
REGULARITY 😃 😐 ☹️
MOOD 😃 😐 ☹️
BRAIN CLARITY 😃 😐 ☹️

Journaling

....
....
....
....
....
....
....
....
....
....
....
....
....

J F M A M J J A S O N D

1 2 3 4 5 6 7 8 9 10 11 12 13 14 15 16

17 18 19 20 21 22 23 24 25 26 27 28 29 30 31 ♥

Fasting Day? YES / NO

FIRST BITE: _____   FASTING HOURS: _____

LAST BITE: _____   EATING HOURS: _____

Sleep

TO BED: _____   HOURS SLEPT: _____

WOKE UP: _____   QUALITY: _____

Food	Time	Note

Exercise	Time	Note

Habits

WATER ⬭ ⬭ ⬭ ⬭ ⬭ ⬭ ⬭

ENERGY LEVEL 😃 😐 ☹️
HUNGER 😃 😐 ☹️
MENTAL STRENGTH 😃 😐 ☹️
REGULARITY 😃 😐 ☹️
MOOD 😃 😐 ☹️
BRAIN CLARITY 😃 😐 ☹️

Journaling

....
....
....
....
....
....
....
....
....
....
....
....
....

Fasting Day? YES / NO

FIRST BITE: _____   FASTING HOURS: _____

LAST BITE: _____   EATING HOURS: _____

Sleep

TO BED: _____   HOURS SLEPT: _____

WOKE UP: _____   QUALITY: _____

Food	Time	Note

Exercise	Time	Note

Habits

WATER ⬨ ⬨ ⬨ ⬨ ⬨ ⬨ ⬨ ⬨

ENERGY LEVEL 😊 😐 ☹️
HUNGER 😊 😐 ☹️
MENTAL STRENGTH 😊 😐 ☹️
REGULARITY 😊 😐 ☹️
MOOD 😊 😐 ☹️
BRAIN CLARITY 😊 😐 ☹️

Journaling

....
....
....
....
....
....
....
....
....
....
....
....
....

| J | F | M | A | M | J | J | A | S | O | N | D |

1 2 3 4 5 6 7 8 9 10 11 12 13 14 15 16

17 18 19 20 21 22 23 24 25 26 27 28 29 30 31 ❤

Fasting Day? YES / NO

FIRST BITE: _____   FASTING HOURS: _____

LAST BITE: _____   EATING HOURS: _____

Sleep

TO BED: _____   HOURS SLEPT: _____

WOKE UP: _____   QUALITY: _____

Food	Time	Note

Exercise	Time	Note

Habits

WATER ⬠ ⬠ ⬠ ⬠ ⬠ ⬠ ⬠ ⬠

ENERGY LEVEL 🙂 😐 🙁
HUNGER 🙂 😐 🙁
MENTAL STRENGTH 🙂 😐 🙁
REGULARITY 🙂 😐 🙁
MOOD 🙂 😐 🙁
BRAIN CLARITY 🙂 😐 🙁

Journaling

....
....
....
....
....
....
....
....
....
....
....
....

(J) (F) (M) (A) (M) (J) (J) (A) (S) (O) (N) (D)

1 2 3 4 5 6 7 8 9 10 11 12 13 14 15 16

17 18 19 20 21 22 23 24 25 26 27 28 29 30 31 ♥

Fasting Day? YES / NO

FIRST BITE: _____   FASTING HOURS: _____

LAST BITE: _____   EATING HOURS: _____

Sleep

TO BED: _____   HOURS SLEPT: _____

WOKE UP: _____   QUALITY: _____

Food	Time	Note

Exercise	Time	Note

Habits

WATER   ⬡ ⬡ ⬡ ⬡ ⬡ ⬡ ⬡

ENERGY LEVEL   🙂 😐 🙁
HUNGER   🙂 😐 🙁
MENTAL STRENGTH   🙂 😐 🙁
REGULARITY   🙂 😐 🙁
MOOD   🙂 😐 🙁
BRAIN CLARITY   🙂 😐 🙁

Journaling

....
....
....
....
....
....
....
....
....
....
....
....

| 1 | 2 | 3 | 4 | 5 | 6 | 7 | 8 | 9 | 10 | 11 | 12 | 13 | 14 | 15 | 16 |

| 17 | 18 | 19 | 20 | 21 | 22 | 23 | 24 | 25 | 26 | 27 | 28 | 29 | 30 | 31 | ♥ |

Fasting Day? YES / NO

FIRST BITE: _____   FASTING HOURS: _____

LAST BITE: _____   EATING HOURS: _____

Sleep

TO BED: _____   HOURS SLEPT: _____

WOKE UP: _____   QUALITY: _____

Food	Time	Note

Exercise	Time	Note

Habits

WATER ⬡⬡⬡⬡⬡⬡⬡⬡

ENERGY LEVEL 😃 😐 ☹️
HUNGER 😃 😐 ☹️
MENTAL STRENGTH 😃 😐 ☹️
REGULARITY 😃 😐 ☹️
MOOD 😃 😐 ☹️
BRAIN CLARITY 😃 😐 ☹️

Journaling

....
....
....
....
....
....
....
....
....
....
....
....
....

Fasting Day? YES / NO

FIRST BITE: _____   FASTING HOURS: _____

LAST BITE: _____   EATING HOURS: _____

Sleep

TO BED: _____   HOURS SLEPT: _____

WOKE UP: _____   QUALITY: _____

Food	Time	Note

Exercise	Time	Note

Habits

WATER ⬭⬭⬭⬭⬭⬭⬭

ENERGY LEVEL ☺ 😐 ☹
HUNGER ☺ 😐 ☹
MENTAL STRENGTH ☺ 😐 ☹
REGULARITY ☺ 😐 ☹
MOOD ☺ 😐 ☹
BRAIN CLARITY ☺ 😐 ☹

Journaling

....
....
....
....
....
....
....
....
....
....
....
....
....

Planning

	S	M	T	W	T	F	S	NOTES
MIDNIGHT								
1:00 AM								
2:00 AM								
3:00 AM								
4:00 AM								
5:00 AM								
6:00 AM								
7:00 AM								
8:00 AM								
9:00 AM								
10:00 AM								
11:00 AM								
NOON								
1:00 PM								
2:00 PM								
3:00 PM								
4:00 PM								
5:00 PM								
6:00 PM								
7:00 PM								
8:00 PM								
9:00 PM								
10:00 PM								
11:00 PM								
MIDNIGHT								

☐ EATING ☐ FASTING ▨ SLEEPING

plan your week
COLOR CODE YOUR HOURS

Fasting Day? YES / NO

FIRST BITE: _____   FASTING HOURS: _____

LAST BITE: _____   EATING HOURS: _____

Sleep

TO BED: _____   HOURS SLEPT: _____

WOKE UP: _____   QUALITY: _____

Food	Time	Note

Exercise	Time	Note

Habits

WATER ⬭⬭⬭⬭⬭⬭⬭⬭

ENERGY LEVEL 😃 😐 ☹️
HUNGER 😃 😐 ☹️
MENTAL STRENGTH 😃 😐 ☹️
REGULARITY 😃 😐 ☹️
MOOD 😃 😐 ☹️
BRAIN CLARITY 😃 😐 ☹️

Journaling

....
....
....
....
....
....
....
....
....
....
....
....

(J) (F) (M) (A) (M) (J) (J) (A) (S) (O) (N) (D)

| 1 | 2 | 3 | 4 | 5 | 6 | 7 | 8 | 9 | 10 | 11 | 12 | 13 | 14 | 15 | 16 |

| 17 | 18 | 19 | 20 | 21 | 22 | 23 | 24 | 25 | 26 | 27 | 28 | 29 | 30 | 31 | ♥ |

Fasting Day? YES / NO

FIRST BITE: _____   FASTING HOURS: _____

LAST BITE: _____   EATING HOURS: _____

Sleep

TO BED: _____   HOURS SLEPT: _____

WOKE UP: _____   QUALITY: _____

Food	Time	Note

Exercise	Time	Note

Habits

WATER ⬡⬡⬡⬡⬡⬡⬡

ENERGY LEVEL ☺ 😐 ☹
HUNGER ☺ 😐 ☹
MENTAL STRENGTH ☺ 😐 ☹
REGULARITY ☺ 😐 ☹
MOOD ☺ 😐 ☹
BRAIN CLARITY ☺ 😐 ☹

Journaling

....
....
....
....
....
....
....
....
....
....
....
....

$\textcircled{J}$ $\textcircled{F}$ $\textcircled{M}$ $\textcircled{A}$ $\textcircled{M}$ $\textcircled{J}$ $\textcircled{J}$ $\textcircled{A}$ $\textcircled{S}$ $\textcircled{O}$ $\textcircled{N}$ $\textcircled{D}$

1 2 3 4 5 6 7 8 9 10 11 12 13 14 15 16

17 18 19 20 21 22 23 24 25 26 27 28 29 30 31 ❤

Fasting Day? YES / NO

FIRST BITE: _____   FASTING HOURS: _____

LAST BITE: _____   EATING HOURS: _____

Sleep

TO BED: _____   HOURS SLEPT: _____

WOKE UP: _____   QUALITY: _____

Food	Time	Note

Exercise	Time	Note

Habits

WATER ◇ ◇ ◇ ◇ ◇ ◇ ◇

ENERGY LEVEL ☺ ☻ ☹
HUNGER ☺ ☻ ☹
MENTAL STRENGTH ☺ ☻ ☹
REGULARITY ☺ ☻ ☹
MOOD ☺ ☻ ☹
BRAIN CLARITY ☺ ☻ ☹

Journaling

....
....
....
....
....
....
....
....
....
....
....
....
....

J F M A M J J A S O N D

| 1 | 2 | 3 | 4 | 5 | 6 | 7 | 8 | 9 | 10 | 11 | 12 | 13 | 14 | 15 | 16 |

17 18 19 20 21 22 23 24 25 26 27 28 29 30 31 ♥

Fasting Day? YES / NO

FIRST BITE: _____   FASTING HOURS: _____

LAST BITE: _____   EATING HOURS: _____

Sleep

TO BED: _____   HOURS SLEPT: _____

WOKE UP: _____   QUALITY: _____

Food	Time	Note

Exercise	Time	Note

Habits

WATER ⬡⬡⬡⬡⬡⬡⬡

ENERGY LEVEL 😀 😐 😟
HUNGER 😀 😐 😟
MENTAL STRENGTH 😀 😐 😟
REGULARITY 😀 😐 😟
MOOD 😀 😐 😟
BRAIN CLARITY 😀 😐 😟

Journaling

....
....
....
....
....
....
....
....
....
....
....
....
....

Fasting Day? YES / NO

FIRST BITE: _____   FASTING HOURS: _____

LAST BITE: _____   EATING HOURS: _____

Sleep

TO BED: _____   HOURS SLEPT: _____

WOKE UP: _____   QUALITY: _____

Food	Time	Note

Exercise	Time	Note

Habits

WATER ⬡ ⬡ ⬡ ⬡ ⬡ ⬡ ⬡

ENERGY LEVEL 😀 😐 🙁
HUNGER 😀 😐 🙁
MENTAL STRENGTH 😀 😐 🙁
REGULARITY 😀 😐 🙁
MOOD 😀 😐 🙁
BRAIN CLARITY 😀 😐 🙁

Journaling

....
....
....
....
....
....
....
....
....
....
....
....
....

| J | F | M | A | M | J | J | A | S | O | N | D |

1 2 3 4 5 6 7 8 9 10 11 12 13 14 15 16

17 18 19 20 21 22 23 24 25 26 27 28 29 30 31 ♥

Fasting Day? YES / NO

FIRST BITE: _____   FASTING HOURS: _____

LAST BITE: _____   EATING HOURS: _____

Sleep

TO BED: _____   HOURS SLEPT: _____

WOKE UP: _____   QUALITY: _____

Food	Time	Note

Exercise	Time	Note

Habits

WATER ⬡ ⬡ ⬡ ⬡ ⬡ ⬡ ⬡ ⬡

ENERGY LEVEL 😊 😐 ☹️
HUNGER 😊 😐 ☹️
MENTAL STRENGTH 😊 😐 ☹️
REGULARITY 😊 😐 ☹️
MOOD 😊 😐 ☹️
BRAIN CLARITY 😊 😐 ☹️

Journaling

....
....
....
....
....
....
....
....
....
....
....
....

(J) (F) (M) (A) (M) (J) (J) (A) (S) (O) (N) (D)

1 2 3 4 5 6 7 8 9 10 11 12 13 14 15 16

17 18 19 20 21 22 23 24 25 26 27 28 29 30 31 ♥

Fasting Day? YES / NO

FIRST BITE: _____   FASTING HOURS: _____

LAST BITE: _____   EATING HOURS: _____

Sleep

TO BED: _____   HOURS SLEPT: _____

WOKE UP: _____   QUALITY: _____

Food	Time	Note

Exercise	Time	Note

Habits

WATER ⬦⬦⬦⬦⬦⬦⬦⬦

ENERGY LEVEL ☺ ☺ ☹
HUNGER ☺ ☺ ☹
MENTAL STRENGTH ☺ ☺ ☹
REGULARITY ☺ ☺ ☹
MOOD ☺ ☺ ☹
BRAIN CLARITY ☺ ☺ ☹

Journaling

....
....
....
....
....
....
....
....
....
....
....
....
....

Planning

	S	M	T	W	T	F	S	NOTES
MIDNIGHT								....
1:00 AM								....
2:00 AM								....
3:00 AM								....
4:00 AM								....
5:00 AM								....
6:00 AM								....
7:00 AM								....
8:00 AM								....
9:00 AM								....
10:00 AM								....
11:00 AM								....
NOON								....
1:00 PM								....
2:00 PM								....
3:00 PM								....
4:00 PM								....
5:00 PM								....
6:00 PM								....
7:00 PM								....
8:00 PM								....
9:00 PM								....
10:00 PM								....
11:00 PM								....
MIDNIGHT								....
								....

☐ EATING   ☐ FASTING   ▨ SLEEPING

plan your week
COLOR CODE YOUR HOURS

Fasting Day? YES / NO

FIRST BITE: _____   FASTING HOURS: _____

LAST BITE: _____   EATING HOURS: _____

Sleep

TO BED: _____   HOURS SLEPT: _____

WOKE UP: _____   QUALITY: _____

Food	Time	Note

Exercise	Time	Note

Habits

WATER ⬡ ⬡ ⬡ ⬡ ⬡ ⬡ ⬡

ENERGY LEVEL 😄 😐 🙁
HUNGER 😄 😐 🙁
MENTAL STRENGTH 😄 😐 🙁
REGULARITY 😄 😐 🙁
MOOD 😄 😐 🙁
BRAIN CLARITY 😄 😐 🙁

Journaling

....
....
....
....
....
....
....
....
....
....
....
....
....

Fasting Day? YES / NO

FIRST BITE: _____   FASTING HOURS: _____

LAST BITE: _____   EATING HOURS: _____

Sleep

TO BED: _____   HOURS SLEPT: _____

WOKE UP: _____   QUALITY: _____

Food	Time	Note

Exercise	Time	Note

Habits

WATER ⬡ ⬡ ⬡ ⬡ ⬡ ⬡ ⬡

ENERGY LEVEL 😃 😐 🙁

HUNGER 😃 😐 🙁

MENTAL STRENGTH 😃 😐 🙁

REGULARITY 😃 😐 🙁

MOOD 😃 😐 🙁

BRAIN CLARITY 😃 😐 🙁

Journaling

....

....

....

....

....

....

....

....

....

....

....

....

....

Fasting Day? YES / NO

FIRST BITE: _____   FASTING HOURS: _____

LAST BITE: _____   EATING HOURS: _____

Sleep

TO BED: _____   HOURS SLEPT: _____

WOKE UP: _____   QUALITY: _____

Food	Time	Note

Exercise	Time	Note

Habits

WATER ⬡ ⬡ ⬡ ⬡ ⬡ ⬡ ⬡

ENERGY LEVEL 🙂 😐 🙁
HUNGER 🙂 😐 🙁
MENTAL STRENGTH 🙂 😐 🙁
REGULARITY 🙂 😐 🙁
MOOD 🙂 😐 🙁
BRAIN CLARITY 🙂 😐 🙁

Journaling

....
....
....
....
....
....
....
....
....
....
....
....
....

Fasting Day? YES / NO

FIRST BITE: _____   FASTING HOURS: _____

LAST BITE: _____   EATING HOURS: _____

Sleep

TO BED: _____   HOURS SLEPT: _____

WOKE UP: _____   QUALITY: _____

Food	Time	Note

Exercise	Time	Note

Habits

WATER ⬡ ⬡ ⬡ ⬡ ⬡ ⬡ ⬡

ENERGY LEVEL ☺ 😐 ☹
HUNGER ☺ 😐 ☹
MENTAL STRENGTH ☺ 😐 ☹
REGULARITY ☺ 😐 ☹
MOOD ☺ 😐 ☹
BRAIN CLARITY ☺ 😐 ☹

Journaling

....
....
....
....
....
....
....
....
....
....
....
....
....

Fasting Day? YES / NO

FIRST BITE: _____   FASTING HOURS: _____

LAST BITE: _____   EATING HOURS: _____

Sleep

TO BED: _____   HOURS SLEPT: _____

WOKE UP: _____   QUALITY: _____

Food	Time	Note

Exercise	Time	Note

Habits

WATER ⬡ ⬡ ⬡ ⬡ ⬡ ⬡ ⬡ ⬡

ENERGY LEVEL 😄 😐 ☹️
HUNGER 😄 😐 ☹️
MENTAL STRENGTH 😄 😐 ☹️
REGULARITY 😄 😐 ☹️
MOOD 😄 😐 ☹️
BRAIN CLARITY 😄 😐 ☹️

Journaling

....
....
....
....
....
....
....
....
....
....
....
....
....

Fasting Day? YES / NO

FIRST BITE: _____   FASTING HOURS: _____

LAST BITE: _____   EATING HOURS: _____

Sleep

TO BED: _____   HOURS SLEPT: _____

WOKE UP: _____   QUALITY: _____

Food	Time	Note

Exercise	Time	Note

Habits

WATER ◇◇◇◇◇◇◇

ENERGY LEVEL	☺ ☺ ☹
HUNGER	☺ ☺ ☹
MENTAL STRENGTH	☺ ☺ ☹
REGULARITY	☺ ☺ ☹
MOOD	☺ ☺ ☹
BRAIN CLARITY	☺ ☺ ☹

Journaling

....

....

....

....

....

....

....

....

....

....

....

....

....

Fasting Day? YES / NO

FIRST BITE: _____   FASTING HOURS: _____

LAST BITE: _____   EATING HOURS: _____

Sleep

TO BED: _____   HOURS SLEPT: _____

WOKE UP: _____   QUALITY: _____

Food	Time	Note

Exercise	Time	Note

Habits

WATER ◊ ◊ ◊ ◊ ◊ ◊ ◊

ENERGY LEVEL ☺ ☺ ☹
HUNGER ☺ ☺ ☹
MENTAL STRENGTH ☺ ☺ ☹
REGULARITY ☺ ☺ ☹
MOOD ☺ ☺ ☹
BRAIN CLARITY ☺ ☺ ☹

Journaling

....
....
....
....
....
....
....
....
....
....
....
....
....

Planning

	S	M	T	W	T	F	S	NOTES
MIDNIGHT								
1:00 AM								....
2:00 AM								....
3:00 AM								....
4:00 AM								....
5:00 AM								....
6:00 AM								....
7:00 AM								....
8:00 AM								....
9:00 AM								....
10:00 AM								....
11:00 AM								....
NOON								....
1:00 PM								....
2:00 PM								....
3:00 PM								....
4:00 PM								....
5:00 PM								....
6:00 PM								....
7:00 PM								....
8:00 PM								....
9:00 PM								....
10:00 PM								....
11:00 PM								....
MIDNIGHT								....

☐ EATING   ☐ FASTING   ☒ SLEEPING

plan your week
COLOR CODE YOUR HOURS

Fasting Day? YES / NO

FIRST BITE: _____   FASTING HOURS: _____

LAST BITE: _____   EATING HOURS: _____

Sleep

TO BED: _____   HOURS SLEPT: _____

WOKE UP: _____   QUALITY: _____

Food	Time	Note

Exercise	Time	Note

Habits

WATER ⬡ ⬡ ⬡ ⬡ ⬡ ⬡ ⬡

ENERGY LEVEL ☺ 😐 ☹
HUNGER ☺ 😐 ☹
MENTAL STRENGTH ☺ 😐 ☹
REGULARITY ☺ 😐 ☹
MOOD ☺ 😐 ☹
BRAIN CLARITY ☺ 😐 ☹

Journaling

....

....

....

....

....

....

....

....

....

....

....

....

....

Fasting Day? YES / NO

FIRST BITE: _____   FASTING HOURS: _____

LAST BITE: _____   EATING HOURS: _____

Sleep

TO BED: _____   HOURS SLEPT: _____

WOKE UP: _____   QUALITY: _____

Food	Time	Note

Exercise	Time	Note

Habits

WATER ⬡ ⬡ ⬡ ⬡ ⬡ ⬡ ⬡

ENERGY LEVEL 😃 😐 ☹️
HUNGER 😃 😐 ☹️
MENTAL STRENGTH 😃 😐 ☹️
REGULARITY 😃 😐 ☹️
MOOD 😃 😐 ☹️
BRAIN CLARITY 😃 😐 ☹️

Journaling

....
....
....
....
....
....
....
....
....
....
....
....
....

Fasting Day? YES / NO

FIRST BITE: _____   FASTING HOURS: _____

LAST BITE: _____   EATING HOURS: _____

Sleep

TO BED: _____   HOURS SLEPT: _____

WOKE UP: _____   QUALITY: _____

Food	Time	Note

Exercise	Time	Note

Habits

WATER ⬡⬡⬡⬡⬡⬡⬡

ENERGY LEVEL ☻ ☺ ☹
HUNGER ☻ ☺ ☹
MENTAL STRENGTH ☻ ☺ ☹
REGULARITY ☻ ☺ ☹
MOOD ☻ ☺ ☹
BRAIN CLARITY ☻ ☺ ☹

Journaling

....
....
....
....
....
....
....
....
....
....
....
....
....

Fasting Day? YES / NO

FIRST BITE: _____   FASTING HOURS: _____

LAST BITE: _____   EATING HOURS: _____

Sleep

TO BED: _____   HOURS SLEPT: _____

WOKE UP: _____   QUALITY: _____

Food	Time	Note

Exercise	Time	Note

Habits

WATER   ⬦ ⬦ ⬦ ⬦ ⬦ ⬦ ⬦

ENERGY LEVEL   😊 😐 ☹️
HUNGER   😊 😐 ☹️
MENTAL STRENGTH   😊 😐 ☹️
REGULARITY   😊 😐 ☹️
MOOD   😊 😐 ☹️
BRAIN CLARITY   😊 😐 ☹️

Journaling

....
....
....
....
....
....
....
....
....
....
....
....

(J) (F) (M) (A) (M) (J) (J) (A) (S) (O) (N) (D)

| 1 | 2 | 3 | 4 | 5 | 6 | 7 | 8 | 9 | 10 | 11 | 12 | 13 | 14 | 15 | 16 |

17 18 19 20 21 22 23 24 25 26 27 28 29 30 31 ♥

Fasting Day? YES / NO

FIRST BITE: _____   FASTING HOURS: _____

LAST BITE: _____   EATING HOURS: _____

Sleep

TO BED: _____   HOURS SLEPT: _____

WOKE UP: _____   QUALITY: _____

Food	Time	Note

Exercise	Time	Note

Habits

WATER   ⬡ ⬡ ⬡ ⬡ ⬡ ⬡ ⬡

ENERGY LEVEL ☺ 😐 ☹
HUNGER ☺ 😐 ☹
MENTAL STRENGTH ☺ 😐 ☹
REGULARITY ☺ 😐 ☹
MOOD ☺ 😐 ☹
BRAIN CLARITY ☺ 😐 ☹

Journaling

....
....
....
....
....
....
....
....
....
....
....
....

Fasting Day? YES / NO

FIRST BITE: _____   FASTING HOURS: _____

LAST BITE: _____   EATING HOURS: _____

Sleep

TO BED: _____   HOURS SLEPT: _____

WOKE UP: _____   QUALITY: _____

Food	Time	Note

Exercise	Time	Note

Habits

WATER ⬭⬭⬭⬭⬭⬭⬭

ENERGY LEVEL 😃 😐 🙁
HUNGER 😃 😐 🙁
MENTAL STRENGTH 😃 😐 🙁
REGULARITY 😃 😐 🙁
MOOD 😃 😐 🙁
BRAIN CLARITY 😃 😐 🙁

Journaling

....
....
....
....
....
....
....
....
....
....
....
....
....

Fasting Day? YES / NO

FIRST BITE: _____   FASTING HOURS: _____

LAST BITE: _____   EATING HOURS: _____

Sleep

TO BED: _____   HOURS SLEPT: _____

WOKE UP: _____   QUALITY: _____

Food	Time	Note

Exercise	Time	Note

Habits

WATER ⬡ ⬡ ⬡ ⬡ ⬡ ⬡ ⬡

ENERGY LEVEL 😀 😐 🙁
HUNGER 😀 😐 🙁
MENTAL STRENGTH 😀 😐 🙁
REGULARITY 😀 😐 🙁
MOOD 😀 😐 🙁
BRAIN CLARITY 😀 😐 🙁

Journaling

....
....
....
....
....
....
....
....
....
....
....
....
....

Made in the USA
Monee, IL
23 May 2021